Praise for *Natural Childbirth Exercise Essentials*

Rhondda is the pioneer leader in the dawning of a new era of drug-free childbirth, appropriately called Natural Childbirth.

Robert A. Bradley, A.B., M.D. (1917-1998)
Founder, American Academy of
Husband-Coached Childbirth®

As I worked side-by-side with my beloved step-father, Dr. Robert Bradley, the amazing effect Rhondda Hartman had on our patients was proven daily with the successful outcomes of thousands of births. Get *Natural Childbirth Exercise Essentials*—for yourself and any one you know who is pregnant.

Susan Lindemann Nelson

With great enthusiasm, I highly commend the exercises and teachings of Rhondda Hartman. Does it make a difference? Indeed! *Natural Childbirth Exercise Essentials* is long overdue.

Max D. Bartlett, MD
former partner of Robert A. Bradley, MD

Get *Natural Childbirth Exercise Essentials*—if you are pregnant, if you are the spouse or partner of a pregnant woman or if you are a health care provider. Any and all will benefit from learning about and using these exercises that will ease the birth for both baby and mother.

Mary Ann Kerwin
Co-Founder of La Leche League International

Rhondda's classes and exercises prepared me beautifully for my son's birth. Her relaxing techniques really work! Read this book, practice her exercises, use her wisdom. It is all there in *Natural Childbirth Exercise Essentials*.

Roberta Scaer, co-author
Good Birth, Safe Birth

If you are imagining heaving, sweating routines—no worries. Some of the exercises aren't even "exercises"! Many are simply "postures" any woman can practice pregnant, and throughout their lives, to maintain strength and flexibility.

Allie Chee, author
New Mother

With Rhondda Hartman's *Natural Childbirth Exercise Essentials*, anyone can access reliable, accurate and proven tips, techniques and exercises to help them prepare for a positive birth experience.

Krystyna Bowman
Bradley Method teacher

Natural Childbirth Exercise Essentials

Rhondda Evans Hartman

Natural Childbirth Exercise Essentials
by Rhondda Evans Hartman

Books may be purchased in bulk or otherwise, by contacting the publisher and author at: RE.Hartman@Live.com.

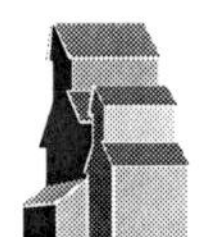

Parkland Press, Ltd.
3755 S. Broadway
Englewood, CO 80110

Cover and Interior Design: Nick Zelinger (NZ Graphics.com)
Book Consultant: Judith Briles, (TheBookShepherd.com)
Sketch Arrtist: Deborah Springer

ISBN: 978-0-9884110-0-5 (print book)
ISBN: 978-0-9884110-1-2 (e-book)

LCCN: 2015917596

1) Childbirth 2) Pregnancy 3) Exercise 4) Women's Health

First Edition Printed in the United States

Dedicated
to all Mothers
who choose Natural Childbirth
because you want only the best
for your baby.
May it be the best birth ever for you!

Contents

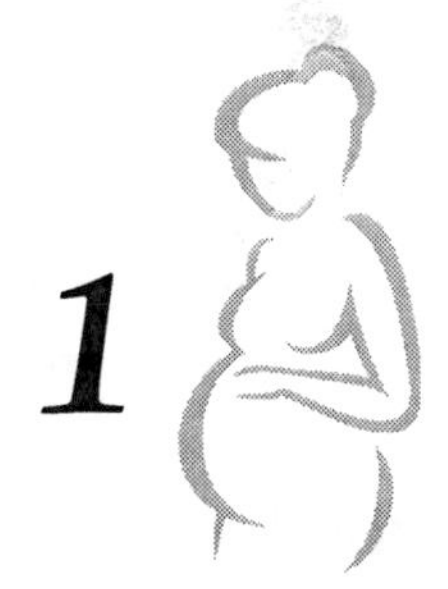

1

Hooray! There is a Baby on the Way ...

I am a mother of five, and cheerleader for over 14,000 mothers and their babies that attended my classes, not to mention the countless numbers who have read my books, *Exercises for True Natural Childbirth* and *Natural Childbirth Exercises: for the Best Birth Ever.* As a pioneer in the Natural Childbirth Movement, I developed these exercises with Dr. Bradley. I am very confident that if you will use the exercises recommended and described and do all the practicing that I tell you to do, you can enjoy your births. I did it and you can, too!

Dr. Bradley and I planned our education of Natural Childbirth as a joint effort for his Medical Obstetric Practice. He gave lectures to the couples to instruct them in the medical aspects of *Husband Coached Childbirth* and I taught the pregnant moms-to-be to prepare themselves mentally, physically and emotionally for the birth.

- I am convinced that everything I taught then is just as valid now as it was then.
- I believe that it is important that you young women of today accept the responsibility of your own bodies, health and especially your own birth.
- No one can do it for you.
- You are the expert.
- You can do it.
- The rewards are stupendous.

- Childbirth is work. Embrace the work.
- You cannot complete any athletic event without hard work.

Birth is an Athletic Event

I suggest you use this book very methodically, *exercise by exercise*, so that you will really have your body and muscles ready by full-term pregnancy. Some of the basic, important postures you need to learn as soon as possible so that you will be comfortable for your whole pregnancy.

Give yourself enough time to be really prepared by the time you have your baby. Do not wait until the last few weeks!

Labor is not easy, it is work, the most wonderful work you will ever do.

However and wherever you give birth, the exercises that you will learn in *Natural Childbirth Exercise Essentials* will greatly enhance your experience for you and your baby.

I was trained as a Registered Nurse so hospital birth is what I know. I am also a Natural Childbirth Educator and know what it takes to have a successful natural birth. I am part of The Bradley Method and am on the Advisory Board of the American Academy of Husband Coached Childbirth. I highly recommend the Bradley Method.

No matter what birth you plan; hospital, birth center, home, epidural or even Cesarean Section ... everything in this book is essential to you. Your physical and mental preparation is necessary no matter where or how you plan to give birth.

Become an Expert

Read everything you can during early pregnancy. Learn about all the various methods and philosophies of childbirth. Find out what is available in your area. Ask, listen, and learn. You may have many options for classes or you may have none. Choose the method or theory and a teacher who most appeals to you.

My choice for you of course is Natural Childbirth with the Bradley Method. Look for truly non-medicated Natural Childbirth instruction which describes the harmful results of medications for the mother and baby. Once you are committed to a class, make sure the philosophy is true Natural Childbirth and make your Birth Plan accordingly. It is vitally important that your baby gets the benefits of an unmedicated birth.

A class setting is a very comfortable way to become an expert in Childbirth. It's fun and social. I recommend you search, visit and find one that appeals to you.

If all else fails and you can't locate a suitable Natural Childbirth Class, I have written two books about this. My second was published recently and I hope you will read it: *Natural Childbirth Exercises for the Best Birth Ever*. It gives much more detail than you will find in this Workbook. I have stories from women who have been able to have joyous successful natural births from using my books. It makes me happy to know that it works!

Natural Childbirth training will be helpful to all, even if you happen to be one who needs medical intervention. Relax and work with your body. There are usually many hours in a labor, even if anesthesia becomes necessary, all your training will be very helpful. The exercises are your guide to a healthy, strong body for your birth and your lifetime.

Have I led you to believe that having a baby is easy? No. Please note, I did not say easy. When you are educated about the work you are undertaking and use the tools that I have given you to enhance it, you will be thrilled by the outcome just as I was with each of my five births.

My hope is that you will accept childbirth for what it is, labor. It is more work going on in your body than you've ever experienced. I hope you will appreciate the forces and be in awe of what is happening during the birth process. If you are well prepared, you will not let those forces overwhelm you, but will work with them to accomplish the goal.

These nine months are a great period in your life. Enjoy and experience them to the fullest.

Happy *Birth* Day!

Rhondda's AHA

May you have a healthy and happy pregnancy and a joyful childbirth!
Check my website, *NaturalChildbirthExercises.com* and find me on
Facebook.com/NaturalChildbirthExercises or Twitter@BirthExercises
for more birth related discussions.

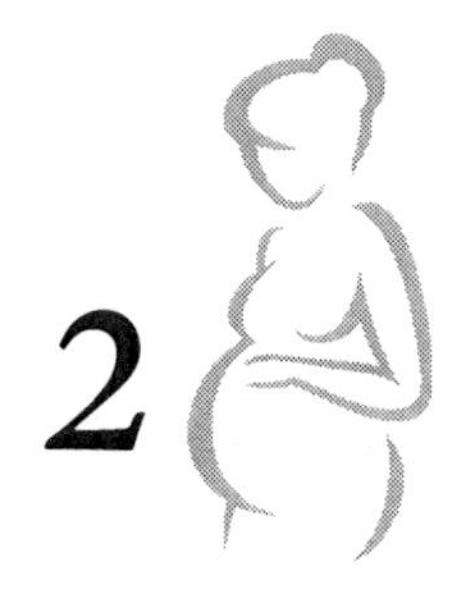

2

Tailor Sit

Not an Exercise, Just a Comfortable Way to Sit

Exercises do not have to be calisthenics. In most cases, Natural Childbirth Exercises are postures and not exercises at all but exercise is an easy word to use. Many of the exercises concentrate on your posture and your daily activities. Do not expect to break into a sweat. Think of this as a very relaxed form of exercise which helps strengthen your body for pregnancy and giving birth.

The goal is to get your body into shape.
You do not compete with anyone.
You do the best you can.

Most of our postures are designed to be used around the home in your everyday activities. Many can be done anywhere you work, but all can easily be fit in if you work at your house all day. Some are to be used for your pregnancy and some prepare you for labor. However, many are to be maintained for the rest of your life.

Do not make yourself stiff and sore by overusing your muscles at first. Begin slowly and I'll give you guidelines in many cases but remember that you are the one who will have the baby. Don't be too easy on yourself but not too hard, either.

Some of the exercises and techniques you will be learning will be for labor but must be learned now and practiced throughout your pregnancy so that you will be good at it when you are in labor. For example, if you haven't practiced enough on your abdominal breathing, it's very hard to learn while in labor. Enlist the help of your husband or your labor coach to remind you. Get a good nine months of training. It will be to your benefit if you are diligent.

Let's begin with our first "exercise"—tailor sitting, an exercise that will add to your comfort as your belly gets bigger.

Tailor Sit

Never stand when you can sit; and when you sit—tailor sit!

Why? For one thing, because tailor sitting is comfortable. Children and many cultures use this position without teaching.

Sitting tailor fashion, with your elbows on your knees, tilts the heavy uterus forward, away from your back and up and out of the pelvis. This teeter-totter effect, with the uterus tilted over the front pelvic bone, allows release of pressure and therefore permits good circulation of blood to the pelvic area, to kidneys, vagina and legs. The blood carries nutrients and oxygen to the uterus and your baby.

Tailor sitting keeps you from sitting in a chair in the usual manner—leaning back and allowing a backward tilt of the uterus—which puts pressure on blood vessels supplying the kidneys, uterus and legs, thereby reducing circulation. Crossing your knees further aggravates the problem and reduces circulation to the vagina.

Tailor sitting stretches and makes flexible the muscles of your bottom and the inner aspects of your thighs, enabling you to put your legs farther apart in second-stage labor, which will be helpful.

It may sound ridiculous, but the effect of increased light and air to your perineum is a healthy extra as it will help prevent vaginal yeast infections.

HOW:

Sit on the floor or any firm surface.
Cross your ankles and bring them close to your body with knees wide apart. You may lean back slightly to reduce the weight on your ankles.
A small pillow under the tail bone will also reduce pressure and may be more comfortable.
This is not an exercise but rather a posture.

Variations:

You may use variations to keep comfortable while sitting for longer periods. As one position becomes crampy, change to a variation:

- Put the soles of your feet together, with knees bent and wide apart, as shown.

OR:

- Stretch and move your feet and legs until you are comfortable, then

- Resume classic Tailor Sit Position.

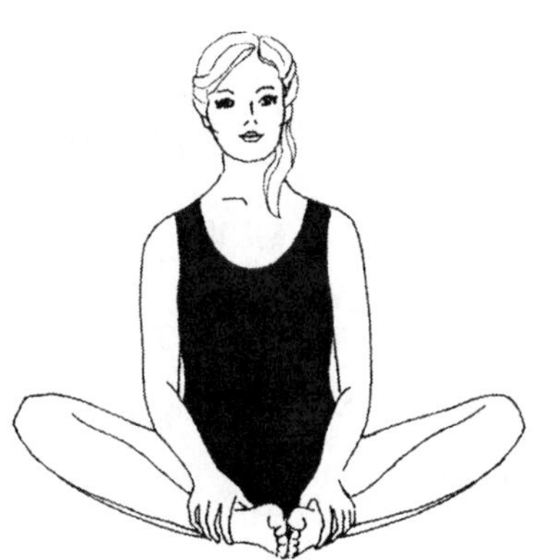

Do not sit in any one position for long periods of time or your legs will go to sleep from lack of good circulation. Even if you sit in a chair, you don't punish yourself by never moving! Most of us find this tailor sitting position easy from all our activities in normal life but if it is difficult for you, rest your elbows on your knees with slight pressure. Do this for short periods. Never make yourself uncomfortable! Don't force your knees to the floor. That is not necessary and may be painful.

After a few weeks, you'll be comfortable for longer periods and your knees will come closer to the floor. Your knees may never touch the floor, since individuals differ. If you are very limber and your knees do touch the floor, this position will be very easy for you to use. You are ahead of most of us in preparation for Natural Childbirth!

WHERE:

Always choose a hard, level surface so that your hips and feet are on the same plane. Tucking a small pillow under your tail bone as you are getting used to this position may be more comfy but as you become good at it you probably will find a padded hard surface such as a carpeted floor much more to your liking.

WHEN:

Anytime you can sit down! For example:

- Reading to the children or yourself.
- Doing needlework, or whatever handicrafts you enjoy.
- Cleaning drawers or lower cupboards (take the drawer out of the chest and put it on the floor).

- Riding in a car, watching television, writing letters, watching movies,
- Eating dinner at a coffee table while sitting on the floor—usually in your own home.
- Playing cards or any games when you can sit on the floor instead of in a chair. Can't you see a foursome playing Scrabble sitting on the floor practicing their tailor sitting?
- During a conversation—sit on the floor, not on the sofa.
- Folding clothes from the dryer.
- With children, tailor sit for everything you do. You will be on their level as you diaper, dress, feed, cuddle, hug, listen, talk, play, fix a hurt, pick up toys—the list is twenty-four hours long!
- You can sit this way in many chairs—from the ordinary hard kitchen chair (you may need a pad for your ankles) to one that is cushy and comfortable.
- What other ways can you think of to use tailor sitting? Be creative.

Sit in the tailor position for short periods or as long as it is comfortable.

You must use a certain amount of good sense in how you begin a new posture or exercise. Do it as often and as long as you like but do be kind to yourself and gradually work up to your optimum.

If tailor sitting is easy for you, it will be used for a more extended period of time than if you find it difficult. However, it should be used with the idea that you are not trying to set a new record. Make it a part of your life—a useful and comfortable addition to your way of doing things which will also contribute to your health.

Rhondda's AHA

Think of tailor sitting as your friend, not as an enemy.

3

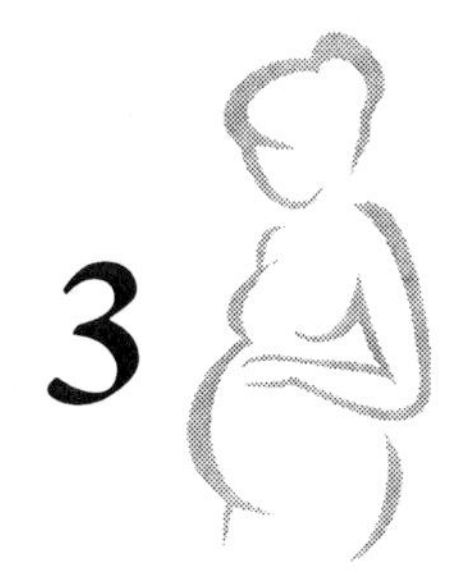

Pelvic Rock for the Rest of your Life

This exercise could be the most important addition to your wellbeing that you have ever learned! It is important to you now during your pregnancy and your birth but it is just as important for the rest of your life.

Dr. Bradley compares us to four footed mammals in *Husband Coached Childbirth* and so we imitate animals in Natural Childbirth with the pelvic rock. And it feels so good! Your uterus and your back will thank you.

As the uterus becomes heavier and heavier with pregnancy, standing upright causes it to push lower and more tightly into the pelvis. This compresses the blood vessels and interferes with circulation to the uterus, legs, and kidneys. The heavy uterus also stretches supportive ligaments that are attached in the small of the back at roughly the same position as in four-footed mammals.

The pressure and the weight cause the pregnant female to "give in" to the uterus, letting it fall forward and sway her back. Backache and pressure pains are the result. Pelvic rocking on hands and knees allows the uterus to fall forward, releasing the pressure in the pelvis and causing no discomfort in the spine because of the all-fours position. In this posture, your spine is a bridge supported on either end by arms and legs.

The rule of Pelvic Rock is this:

When standing hold your spine straight so that the baby is contained in the pelvis.
At regular intervals get on all-fours to do pelvic rocks for the release of pressure in your pelvis. Allowing the uterus to tip out of the pelvis improves circulation to the area but will cause back pain if you do it standing upright.
That is why it is done on all fours!

Pelvic rock will strengthen and tone the muscles in the back and abdomen which will allow you to keep a straight spine and avoid back aches as the uterus pulls on the inside of your back. The uterus is attached by ligaments on the inside of your lower back. As it gets heavier with the baby's growth you need to have very strong muscles in your back along the spine to maintain good posture.

To recap: alternate between a straight back when standing with all fours pelvic rocks to release the uterus and let it hang out!

WHY?

This is an exercise to help you during pregnancy. It strengthens muscles in your back and abdomen and therefore makes it easier for you to carry the baby in your pelvis. These muscles are also involved with the birthing process.

1. Pelvic rocking improves your posture for the rest of your life. This is a lifetime exercise. A straight spine makes you feel and look better whether you are pregnant or not.

2. Pelvic rocking strengthens your back muscles. The muscles along your spine need to be very strong to be able to maintain a straight spine while a heavy uterus is attached to it.

3. Pelvic rocking strengthens abdominal muscles to support the uterus during pregnancy and after the birth.

4. Your tummy will be flatter than ever before.

5. You may even reduce the size and flabbiness of your hips and thighs.

6. Pelvic rocking will help prevent varicose veins by increasing circulation to pelvis and legs. Relieving the pressure of the uterus in the pelvis will relieve pressure on the blood vessels.

7. The relief of pelvic pressure and increased circulation helps prevent hemorrhoids, too.

8. Pelvic rocking increases mobility of the pelvis, which may help in labor as you push the baby through the birth canal.

9. Pelvic rocking will definitely help relieve tensions and relax you in preparation for sleep at night.

HOW:

Get on the floor in an "all-fours" position, making sure that you form a box position. Have your knees and hips in a line and your wrists and shoulders in a line, both of these 'lines' are perpendicular to the floor. Your knees may be comfortably apart.

1. Lower your abdomen toward the floor until you look like a "sway-back horse." (Dr. Bradley's expression!) But only so that you are comfortable. It may be a very small movement.

2. Lift your lower back until your back is parallel with the floor.

3. Tighten buttocks. This raises the back slightly and tightens the abdomen.

4. Slowly return to the "sway-back" position with control.

5. Repeat movements 2 through 4.

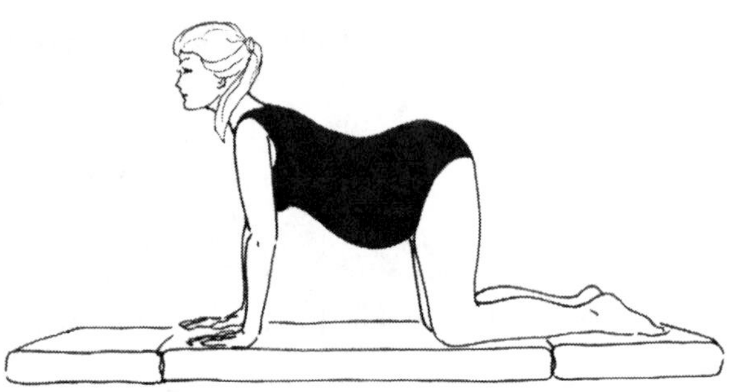

This must be done rhythmically, with as much control lowering as raising the back. It should be done slowly, the whole movement taking about five to seven seconds.

There are a few Dos and Don'ts:

- Do not move your shoulders and upper back. This exercise is for the lower back and pelvis and we ignore the upper back completely.

- It is a different exercise when you raise your upper back and is not specifically helpful in pregnancy or birth.

- Do the cat stretch if you want but I have not included it.

- Do not move your arms either.

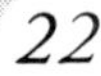

Watching yourself in a mirror while doing this exercise will help you do the movements. Instead of a full-length mirror, try putting a light on the floor to cast your shadow on the wall.

If you develop a pain or a "stitch" in your side as when running, it is a result of dropping your abdomen too quickly or too low. Stop if you feel discomfort and check to see how you are doing the movement. Be cautious with how low your back goes down. Sometimes just tightening the back muscles is all you need to do. It does not have to be a large movement. Use more control and there will be only comfort, never discomfort.

WHERE:

It is very hard to combine this with any other activity in your life.

You will have to get off by yourself several times during the day to do enough pelvic rocks to keep you comfortable. For those of you working outside your homes it is a bit difficult. You might find a ladies' lounge or an unused conference room, a supply room or anyplace where you can get on all fours and do pelvic rocks to relieve the tension in your back.

WHEN:

- Do the pelvic rock the last thing before bed. That is very important.
- Do 80 before bed, with a rest in the middle if you need it.
  Caution: do not start by doing this number. Work up gradually toward the goal of 80 before bed. Try 10 at a time to begin and make sure that you do not make your back stiff and sore by overworking these underused muscles!
- Do at intervals during the day. For example: midmorning, midafternoon, and early evening, 40 each time (start with 10 and increase gradually), then 80 at bedtime.
  I suggest you increase to eighty when you are able to do so comfortably.

After your bedtime pelvic rocks, crawl into bed. Organize your body into the side lying Relaxation position discussed in a later chapter. Now your body is in the perfect posture for the comfort and health of baby and you. You are not lying on the baby nor is the baby's weight resting on you.

Rhondda's AHA

Do extra Pelvic Rocks when you are "too tired to do any."

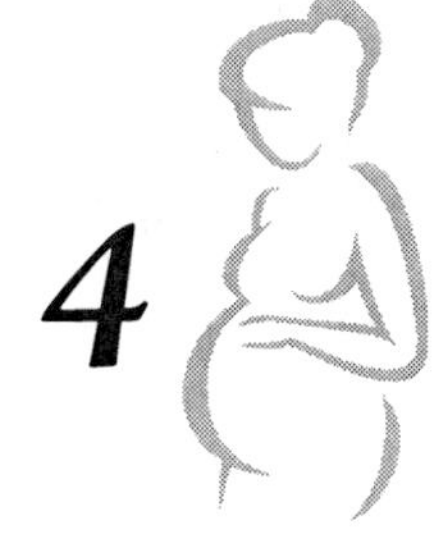

4

Variations of Pelvic Rock, Just for Fun

Since Pelvic Rocking is so vital to your comfort and health during pregnancy, here are some additional positions. The hands-and-knees position is by far the most effective means of "rocking your pelvis," so use it whenever possible.

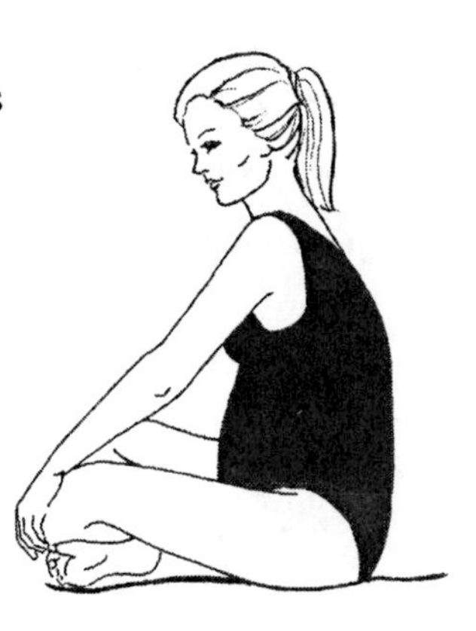

Sitting Pelvic Rock

Though the sitting position is not as effective as the other methods of pelvic rocking, the advantage is that it can be done while you are sitting doing routine tasks. It will relieve back tension and pelvic pressure.

HOW:

1. Begin in a tailor sitting position. Roll your pelvis back so that your weight shifts to the base of your spine. You feel as though you have been pushed in the abdomen.

2. Roll the pelvis forward again as far as it will go. This pushes your abdomen forward.

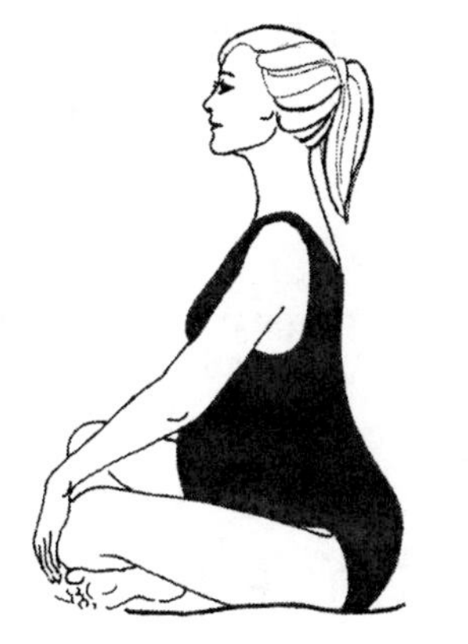

3. After repeating these motions about ten times, stop when the pelvis is level and relaxed.

WHERE:

If you are not able to assume a proper tailor sit position on the floor, you can do the pelvic rock sitting in a chair. Not as effective but helps a bit!

Try to get yourself out of the habit of crossing your legs when sitting in a chair. This contributes to poor circulation and may also help to build "saddlebags" on the sides of your thighs. An even worse possibility is that it could promote varicose veins or hemorrhoids.

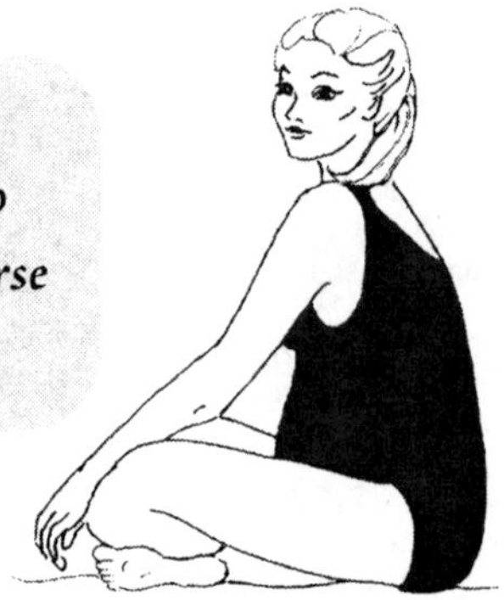

Pelvic rock sitting can be done anywhere: at a desk at the office, at the movies, riding in a car, watching TV, reading, at the computer ... you get the idea. Whenever you are sitting, do occasional pelvic rocks.

WHEN:

Do this mid-morning, noon, mid-afternoon, early evening, and anytime in between. It will be very unobtrusive if done one at a time.

Standing Pelvic Rock

Standing pelvic rock should be learned so well that your posture will improve. Even if you already have perfect posture you will need to strengthen your muscles to maintain it during a pregnancy. Now is a good time to better your postural habits, since you become uncomfortable so easily carrying your growing baby in your uterus. Bad posture will give you a backache. So if you have one, use your pelvic rocks. This exercise will not only prevent backaches, it will ease an aching back, also.

- Standing pelvic rock is especially good for you to build strength in the back muscles so that you can maintain a good posture while standing.
- It makes you look better because it lifts your chin, raises your breasts, pulls your shoulders back, tightens your buttocks, pulls in your abdomen, and unlocks your knees.
- You appear to the world as a woman proud to be having a baby.
- You look and feel two months earlier in pregnancy than you would with a sway-back and a protruding abdomen.
- Standing pelvic rock gives a slight relaxation to the knees and thus aids leg circulation. Varicose vein troubles are decreased.
- If your back is kept straight it will not ache from the weight of the baby tugging on the muscles and ligaments that connect the uterus to your back.
- Some of the stretch of the abdominal wall will be eliminated.
- The amount of loose skin on your abdomen after the baby is born will depend a great deal on how well you have maintained a good posture throughout your pregnancy.
- Add to all this ... it keeps you from walking like a duck!

The baby doesn't ruin your figure—you do!

HOW:

1. Stand facing a chair or any vertical surface. This is only to demonstrate to you how this pelvic rock really makes a difference with your posture.

2. Push your hip and abdomen forward with your tailbone back and up toward the ceiling. Your hand position is not important. Put your hands wherever it is comfortable—shoulders, hips, or down at your side.

3. Now reverse the posture. Tuck your tailbone under you and tighten your buttocks. The top of the pelvis has moved back, bringing the hipbones back, also. Notice how your abdominal wall has tightened and flattened and how much space you now have between your tummy and the chair. Also notice that your knees relax with a slight bend. Keeping them locked and tight will be very uncomfortable

4. Repeat 2 and 3 as many times as you need to make your back feel comfortable.

WHERE and WHEN:

Standing pelvic rock can be done anytime you are standing, such as: waiting in line at the supermarket, waiting to cross the street, when you get out of bed (it will help you get moving in the morning!), every time you look in a mirror, when you get out of a car, getting up after sitting on a sofa, and every time you feel tension in your back.

Obviously, this movement can be done any time you wish or remember to do it. It can become such a habit that you'll do it all day long. Eventually your spine will become permanently straight because the muscles are strong and developed. When you are no longer pregnant you should continue to do this to maintain good posture.

"Kitchen Sink" Pelvic Rock or Mabel Fitzhugh's Pelvic Rock

This exercise was taught to me, personally, by Mabel Lumm Fitzhugh, who shared my passion for Natural Childbirth. She spent several days with me when I was being trained as a new Childbirth Educator.

The "Kitchen Sink" can be anything of the right height—a chair back at the office, the desktop in the schoolroom, a window ledge, bathroom sink, countertop, cupboard, dresser, etc.—wherever you are.

I keep the name because when Mabel taught it, most pregnant women were homemakers and spent lots of time at the kitchen sink. The exercise should be done each time you go to the sink (or to the chair at your desk, etc.). Through frequent practice you will maintain good posture, give yourself quick relief from pelvic pressure, and you will improve circulation to the lower part of your body.

Mrs. Fitzhugh used this exercise as a test on pregnant women in a clinic where no other form of exercise was encouraged. The women showed a marked avoidance of varicose veins and much less back discomfort than a control group.

HOW:

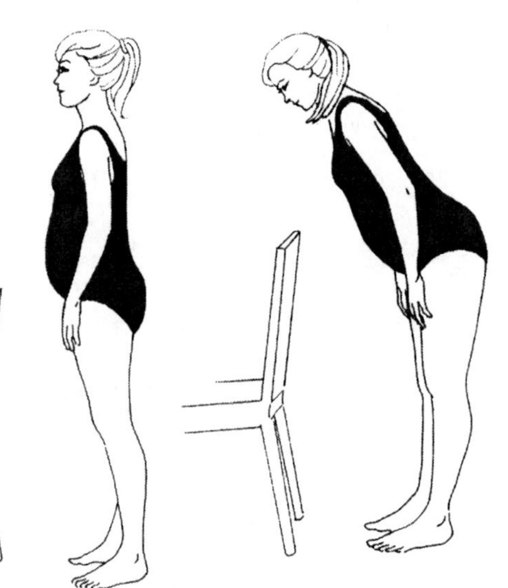

1. Stand straight about two feet away from the sink, with feet comfortably apart (about six inches). Distances will depend upon your size.
2. Bow to the sink! In other words, bend from the hips with a straight back.
3. Put your hands on the edge of the counter, elbows stiff, and let your hands support your weight. That is, lean into your hands.
4. Point your tailbone toward the ceiling. It may hurt behind your knees, so go easy!
5. Tuck your tailbone down and under you, as you relax your knees. This rolls your hipbones backward as your spine gets a comfortable stretch.
6. Do Step 4 and Step 5, three times very slowly.
7. Now, with your lower back rounded, your tailbone tucked under you, knees relaxed, and buttocks tight, straighten your shoulders and head over the rest of your body. Be sure to keep the good posture that you have created in the lower part of your back.

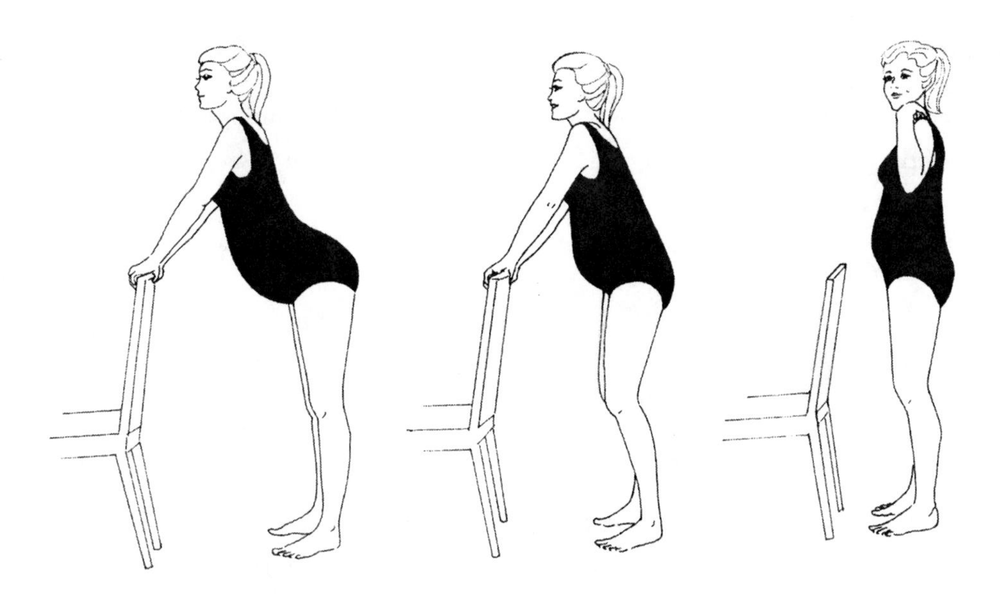

8. Walk up to the counter and find that you can get four inches closer to it! Keep your knees relaxed and the same pelvic posture as you go on to do other things.

9. Repeat each time you go to the sink! Decide what you will use as your "kitchen sink" that will be your reminder to do this often during your busy day.

WHERE:

This can be done at any table, counter, or desk that is the right height for you. If the counter is about the height of the top of your pelvic bone—about two inches below your waist—it is just right.

WHEN:

Do this exercise all day long, every time you go to your kitchen sink—or whatever chair or ledge you decide on as your point of most frequency during the day.

Rhondda's AHA

Knowing about and integrating pelvic rocks in your daily routine will change your physical and mental life. Make pelvic rocks part of your regular routine, just like brushing your teeth.

Why? Simply this: doing pelvic rocks during pregnancy and long after will enhance your life.

Your back muscles will be stronger, your body will look better and you will feel better.

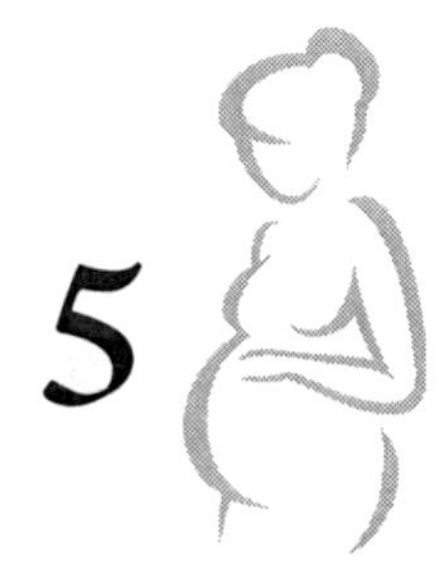

5

Abdominal Breathing

You must become very good at abdominal breathing because during the first stage of labor, with each contraction you will breathe with your abdomen and relax completely. This will allow you to remain comfortable and it will be your secret to having a natural childbirth. Between contractions you may do what you feel like doing and breathe comfortably.

Abdominal breathing and relaxation belong together. You do them better together than you are able to do each separately. Your ability to do both will increase with practice, so the amount of time you spend at it beforehand will pay great dividends during labor.

Learning to relax is a lifetime benefit. It reduces your stress level and increases your vitality.

When you inhale, your abdomen rises—as you exhale, it lowers. The breathing must be very slow and full. Give plenty of time for each part of the breath.

Since your body will be working very hard during labor, you will require great quantities of oxygen to fulfill your needs. At the same time, you must be totally relaxed for your labor to progress smoothly and easily.

Raising the abdominal wall as high as possible is important in labor for another reason. The uterus, as it tightens with a contraction, will bulge. This pushes it against the abdominal wall. Now, if your abdominal muscles are relaxed and being raised slowly with abdominal breathing, there will be minimal discomfort when the contracting, bulging uterus pushes against the abdominal wall. Pull tight on the abdominal muscles and see the tension created between two hard, contracted muscles—the uterus and the abdomen. Make sure you remember this when you are in labor. It is the necessary element in having a natural, comfortable, joyous birth.

Relaxing with abdominal breathing keeps the abdominal muscles soft and relaxed and slowly pushed away from the contracting uterus by your big oxygen-laden inhalation. During exhalation, the abdominal wall along with the whole body remains relaxed to avoid interference with the work of the contracting uterus.

Abdominal Breathing is Necessary

First … you need the large amount of oxygen that this type of deep breathing will allow. Ordinary breathing, usually much more shallow, cannot easily serve the great oxygen needs of the laboring body.

Second … you can relax much better if you breathe in this manner, and only with relaxation will you be comfortable during first-stage labor.

Third … the control used in the breathing helps give you the mastery of your body required to "ride" with each contraction of the uterus. You are the director of this show!

HOW:

1. Sit leaning against a pillow with knees raised to lessen the tension of the abdominal muscles. This position is for learning how, more than for labor. As soon as you have learned the technique, you may practice on your side in a relaxed position.

2. Put your hands low on your abdomen so that you can feel the pubic bone. This guides you to take a deeper breath than if your hands are higher up on the abdomen.

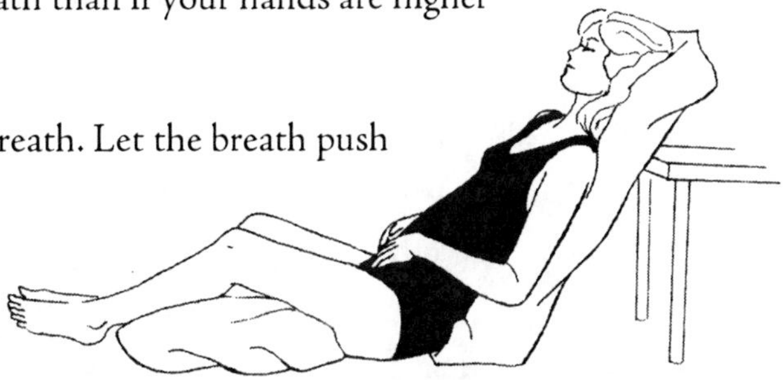

3. Open your mouth and take a deep breath. Let the breath push your abdomen and hands up.

4. Slowly let your breath out and hands and abdomen go down again.

5. Repeat and practice for about two minutes. Breathe slowly and deeply.

6. Now put one hand up on your chest. There should be no chest movement as you continue to breathe abdominally.

Stop and rest! Now do it again, and make each breath as long in duration as is comfortable. Try to "fill your abdomen" with air. Notice the difference between letting the breath push your abdomen up and having the muscles lift your abdomen.

You must not tense your abdominal muscles or any muscles in your body. For you to be comfortable in labor, your abdominal wall must remain relaxed while the uterus is contracting. Sometimes this can be a confusing thing but your husband/coach will be able to feel the difference with his hand and can coach you to know when you are doing well. Practice together now so that you'll be a good team when labor begins.

Dr. Bradley's *Husband-Coached Childbirth* is a good guide for coaching.

WHERE:

Where do you practice? In bed, as you lie down for an afternoon rest (it is a lovely idea, isn't it?) and when you are ready for sleep at night. Do several minutes of concentrated relaxation with abdominal breathing each time.

Begin to use abdominal breathing during the day as you think of it. As you first learn this type of breathing, you may despair that it will ever become easy. It quickly becomes a comfortable way of breathing, though, and by the time you go into labor, it should come very naturally. The more you practice, the easier your first stage of labor will be. When your labor reaches an intensity that demands your attention start relaxing and abdominal breathing with each contraction until the first stage of labor is completed and you are ready to begin pushing.

WHEN:

During pregnancy—Practice often during pregnancy, at least three times each day, taking several breaths. Consider two minutes a good amount of time for a practice contraction, although a contraction would not likely be this long. One minute to one and one-half minutes is more likely, even at transition (end of the first stage).

You will soon learn to breathe abdominally in other positions so that you can practice it all day long. Practice it while sitting in a contour position until you know for sure how to do it, and then alternate with the side-lying relaxation position.

In labor—with each contraction, relax completely and take deep, slow, full abdominal breaths. Continue with abdominal breathing and relaxation for the total time of each contraction. In between you can stretch, move, talk or even go to sleep. With the next contraction, go back to "work" immediately.

Rhondda's AHA

Don't fight this! Practice it often! Any time you have the opportunity to lie down, practice abdominal breathing. As your pregnancy advances and your uterus and belly expand, knowing how to maximize your breathing will not only benefit you overall, it will ease your labor.

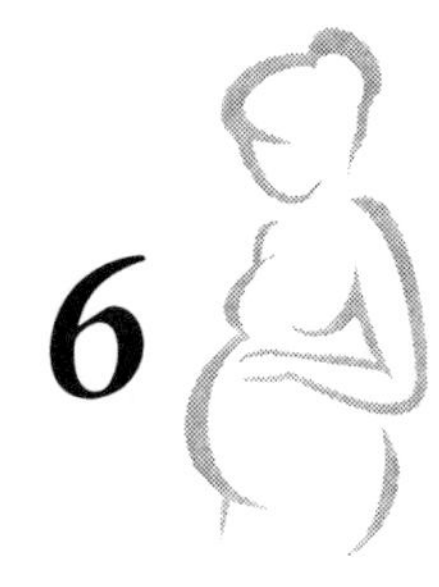

6

Relaxation

The meaning of the word "relaxation" as used in Natural Childbirth may be very different from your past experience. It is a skill that you will find useful for the rest of your life. The benefit of learning and embracing relaxation is actually: ***Let it be! Get out of the way! Do not interfere!***

Here is what the word means to me and to you, too, from now on.

> Relaxation takes mental activity to keep you physically inactive.
> In other words, you work hard with your mind to keep your body
> still and quiet! It is very different from actual sleep, when our minds probably
> fall asleep before our bodies relax. Relaxing takes mental discipline, especially
> while the uterus is in hard contraction.

During relaxation as used in labor, there is absolutely no sleepiness involved but rather a much heightened awareness and complete control over oneself. You may even think of yourself as "working hard" at relaxing.

Remember, it is very passive work physically but hard work mentally.

Relaxation must be considered the most important factor in an enjoyable childbirth experience. *Relaxing is the crux of Natural Childbirth.* The only help you can give the uterus with its work in the first stage of labor is to relax.

Let it be! Get out of the way! Do not interfere!

To do this requires tremendous concentration because the uterus contracts to a hard knot with each contraction. It is a sensation that you can ease your body through if you're relaxed, but what a difference if you are tense! The uterine contraction has many times greater intensity when the muscles surrounding it are also tense and tight.

I've done it five times in childbirth and know that it is so—but you may be skeptical. Each one of you may try it for yourself. It is a very easy theory to prove in labor. Just tighten any group of muscles while you are in the middle of a contraction. For example, make a fist with one hand. You will be convinced that you are having a much harder contraction than you were having previously. It works every time. Try this small experiment while you are in early labor so it will not hurt too much.

You may feel so comfortable you'll not know that your relaxing is responsible for your comfort and that your labor is actually hard. Laughing, coughing, or trying to be polite and answer a nurse or any other activity in the middle of a contraction will prove to you, by contrast, that relaxation works. You will also find out that not doing it right for one contraction does not ruin your whole labor. Just get back into your good relaxing technique and you will have a wonderful experience in your first stage of labor.

In the second stage of labor we do something quite different. Here is my Nutshell explanation of Natural Childbirth. It is my mantra!

Natural Childbirth in a Nutshell

1. In the First Stage of labor, use abdominal breathing and complete relaxation with each contraction.

2. In the Second Stage of labor, take complete, full breaths with each contraction and push as hard as you can while holding your breath.

Just remember that any part of your body in tension is going to add tension to the uterine contraction. That means it will hurt! That is why most people call a contraction a "labor pain." It also detracts from the efficiency of the contracting uterus. That means your labor could be longer. Stay out of the way and let the uterus do its work. You'll feel better and the labor will not be slowed down. And you might never use the word Pain for your labor!

HOW:

1. **Classic Position**—Lie on your side on a firm padded surface with one arm under and behind you, the other bent in front of your face. Both legs are bent at the knee, the upper one pulled forward to help support the weight of your body away from the baby.

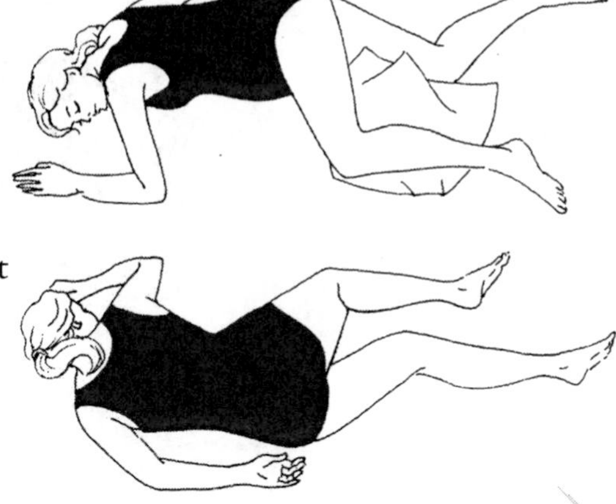

Pillows may be used wherever necessary to make you more comfortable, under your knee, under your leg and foot or under your head and chest to help hold your weight off the lower shoulder or both by using two pillows. Make yourself comfortable.

Every part of your body should be supported. Try putting a pillow under your head then pull the corner of the pillow down between your breasts. If that does not feel good then keep adjusting until it works for you.

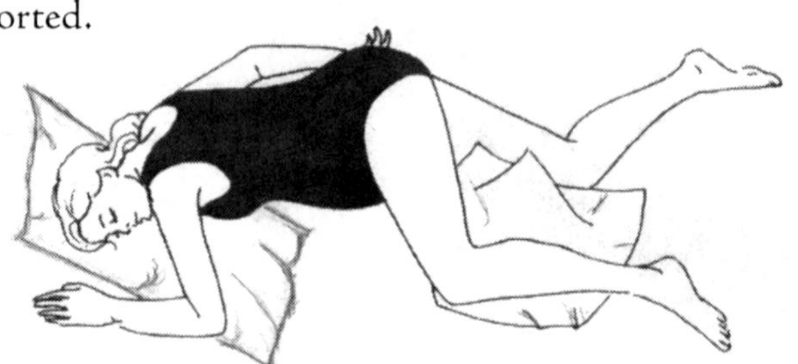

Relaxation is impossible if you are not in a comfortable position as you begin.

2. **Variation of Classic Position**—Your arms may be more comfortable in front, but avoid putting one arm on top of the other or holding your head on your arms, which creates a point of tension.

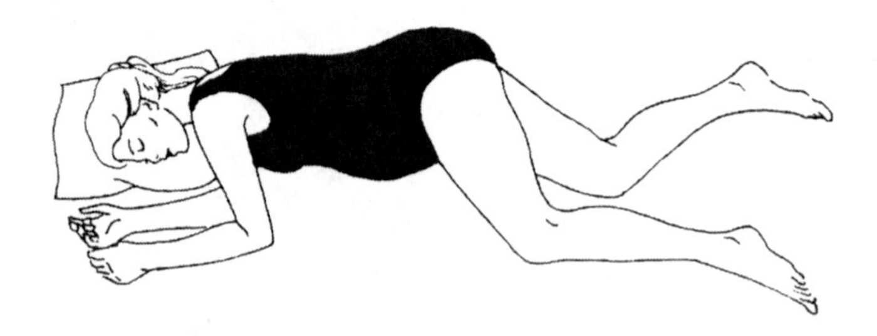

To prepare for relaxation, especially during labor, keep in mind these necessary conditions:

- The proper atmosphere includes absence of strangers, solitude, and a quiet, restful room with as little noise or commotion as possible. Avoid a glaring light, but a soft, dull light will probably be comfortable. Set the stage for this event. Make the environment suit you. It will enhance your relaxation and make your birth an amazingly wonderful experience.

- Use the comfortable positions, as illustrated. These basic positions vary some with each individual. Just make sure that each joint is slightly bent, not straight or fully flexed. Position your body and use pillows to help you become comfortable with all tension relieved. If you are in labor in a hospital, the bed will adjust to help with your positioning. Do not let any one part of the body bear the weight of any other part of the body. In other words, don't have your head resting on your arm, or one leg on the other.

- Control your breathing. Use slow, steady, and relaxed abdominal breathing.

- Complete concentration and attention to what you are doing is imperative. Closing your eyes helps you control your environment. You shut it out and ignore everything!

Get Ready for Loose and Limp!

Now, assume the classic position and get yourself as comfortable and relaxed as you can. If you then have your husband/coach read the poem I've written, you should be able to relax even more. You'll soon observe how you respond to different words and phrases and begin to think creatively about what other words or routines might be better for you. You may prefer to use a "total body" idea of relaxing and not go to the progressive method that I use. Perhaps you will do best with "pleasant thought" or meditative relaxing.

You will benefit in labor if you teach your husband/partner/coach to relax as you are learning the technique. Try it out with whoever is with you. Prove how relaxing it is to speak softly and caringly. Show how hard it is to keep tension in his or her face when you are offering suggestions of a relaxed face. Demonstrate how a bad position will hinder relaxation. Test out words and touching to see what the response is. When your partner learns to relax, he or she will be better able to coach you to perfect relaxation. It is also a good idea for you to see how hard it is to be in the coaching role. You will be a much better team after this reversal of roles.

I offer what I have used effectively for years as a way of easily teaching others to relax—often a very new skill for many people in our fast-living society. So, begin with this and then progress to your own variation. Even if you continue to use my words, you will place your own meaning on them. Relaxing is so personal that I can only teach it the way I feel it. Try to tune in with me and let it work for you.

Whoever you choose to be with you in your pregnancy journey, have him or her read or "croon" this to you slowly and quietly as a poem or a lullaby, giving time for it to take effect:

Loose and Limp . . . Warm and Heavy

Let your whole being
Sink slowly, slowly, slowly.
Feel your muscles
Become limp and loose and comfortable.
Drifting or floating,
Relaxed and comfortable,
warmth and heaviness spread through your body.
The baby in your uterus
is warm and heavy.
Feel warmth and heaviness
spreading from the baby to your abdomen, hips,
thighs, knees, lower legs, ankles,
feet and toes.
Slowly, quietly
the lower half of you is
loose and limp, warm and heavy.
The upper half of you awaits its turn.
Slowly release, let go, warm and heavy,
limp and loose.

Let every cell absorb and enjoy,
spreading up your back and front,

chest and shoulders.
Arms and fingers let go.

As your neck releases tension,
your head slowly shifts and becomes
more and more relaxed.
Nearer and nearer that comfortable state of
relaxation.

Erase the worries from your brow,
eyes loose but closed.
Eyes and all around eyes
limp and loose.
Cheeks loosen and droop,
jaw drops.
Tongue is loose in your mouth,
lips part slightly.
Warm, heavy, and comfortable.
Deep, slow, heavy breathing.
Breathe in and out slowly,
abdomen up and down slowly.
Limp and loose,

warm and heavy,
comfortably relaxed.

In your mind's eye
hold a softly purring kitten in your lap
while sunshine warms you both.
Listen to the laughter of children
sledding on a crisp sparkly snowy hill.
Ride a bicycle on a lazy autumn afternoon,
hair blowing in the wind.
Sit before a roaring, snapping fire
a crisp apple ready to eat.
Watch a robin build her nest,
weaving string and straw with precision.
Lie on the warm sand, you and your love,
while the waves roll up on the beach.

Limp and loose,
warm and heavy,
comfortably relaxed.

WHERE and WHEN:

- **In Labor:** During each contraction in the first stage of labor, you will relax completely and breathe abdominally. In between contractions you will not need to relax but you might fall asleep!
- **Preparing for labor:** will take much practice, so relax whenever you can lie down for a nap and every night as you go to bed. It takes only minutes and will help you relax for sleep.

One good way to test yourself is to spend two minutes on the floor with a soft rug at the busiest time of your day. You may have a toddler pulling at your eyelids and asking, "Are you asleep, Mommy?" That is very good preparation for labor, when you must ignore your environment and concentrate on yourself.

WARNING:
Falling asleep is not good relaxing practice.
You have stopped concentrating on your relaxation or you'd never fall asleep.
So stay awake and focus on the task at hand.

You can relax at other times, too, of course. I do think it best to lie down, but sometimes you could sit in a chair and try to loosen your body as much as possible. Any efforts to relax will help you become better at it.

It works spectacularly with children. Are your children rowdy at bedtime? Just use your relaxing voice and words to calm them down. It's magic!

When I am teaching Relaxing Techniques to groups—some are mothers-to be, their husbands/partners, coaches, Doulas, Midwives, healthcare professionals—anyone who is involved with the care of the mother, it's not uncommon to have multiple little ones crawling around.

Of course they hate it when their mother lies down, closes her eyes and begins to relax. The child feels ignored. For a few minutes there is mild confusion. I begin my soft, crooning relaxing words. The mother will usually put a comforting hand on the child and soon everyone becomes comfortable and quiet. Moms and babies calmly relax. It always works!

During labor you will need to work very hard mentally to keep your body loose and limp all the while your uterus is contracting extremely hard. Your contractions will rarely last more than a minute and two minutes is unusually long. In between contractions you can change position or stretch.

Rhondda's AHA

In very hard labor, you may even fall asleep in between contractions and when the next one wakes you, concentrate on your relaxing and go back to serious abdominal breathing.

7

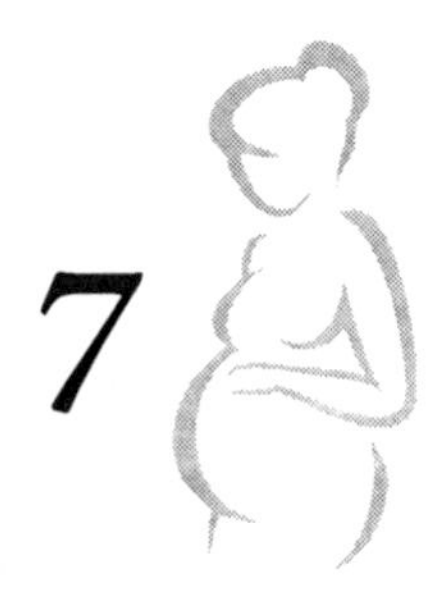

Squatting Makes the Difference

The squat is the position you will assume to give birth. It opens the "baby door," the pelvis is pulled as wide open as it can get. So get busy and limber up those squatting muscles! The wider apart you hold your legs, the sooner the baby can be born.

Squatting is healthy because it develops better circulation in the perineal area, which leads to better muscle tone and healthier tissue. By squatting, you are preparing the perineum to stretch better to allow the birth of your baby. One of the benefits post birth is that your tissues are healthy from the increased attention to them. After the typical stretching that childbirth creates, your tissues are quicker to resume their normal state.

HOW:

Bend your knees as you lower into a squat position, keep your heels on the floor and your toes straight ahead. Keep weight on the outer edges of your feet as much as possible. Place your arms between your knees so that your shoulders and knees are close together.

Use this position only as long as it is comfortable—actually, very short times. Even if you can stay in the squat position for a longer time, be careful, as you may feel "fused" into a squat position before you know it.

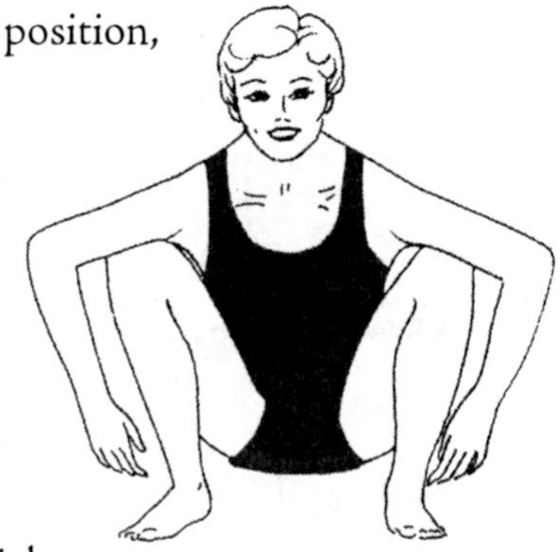

If you cannot balance and you keep falling back into a sitting position, here are some helpful hints.

- Hold on to a heavy object such as the bottom of a chest of drawers, a bed leg, the lower cupboards in the kitchen, the bottom of a closed door—anything that will support your weight and yet keep your hands low enough to maintain a proper squat position.
- It will help you if your clothes are loose or stretchy. You might find it easier to balance while you are learning to squat, if you wear shoes. The bit of a lift from the heel of the shoes will help you balance.
- There is another way to learn to squat by pairing with someone else. Each of you will act as a counter-weight to the other. Grasp your partner's wrists then slowly lower yourselves while at the same time pulling against the bodyweight of your partner. Your back remains straight and your arms are outstretched. Keep lowering yourselves to the squat position. Once you are squatting, maintain it by leaning your shoulders forward between your knees.
- My final suggestion for learning to get into a squat is to stand close to a wall with your back pressed against it. Then slowly slide your back down the wall until you are in a squat. Then you need to find your balance as you lean forward.

If squatting is difficult for you, do not be discouraged. Keep trying, using all these helpful tricks and you will be squatting with ease in no time!

Getting Up from a Squat

HOW:

To come up to a standing position, push your tailbone toward the ceiling as your legs straighten, then raise the upper portion of your body upright. Use your hands on your thighs to help push yourself up. This helps tilt the heavy uterus up and out of the pelvis.

It is a variation of the pelvic rock—think of it as a vertical pelvic rock.

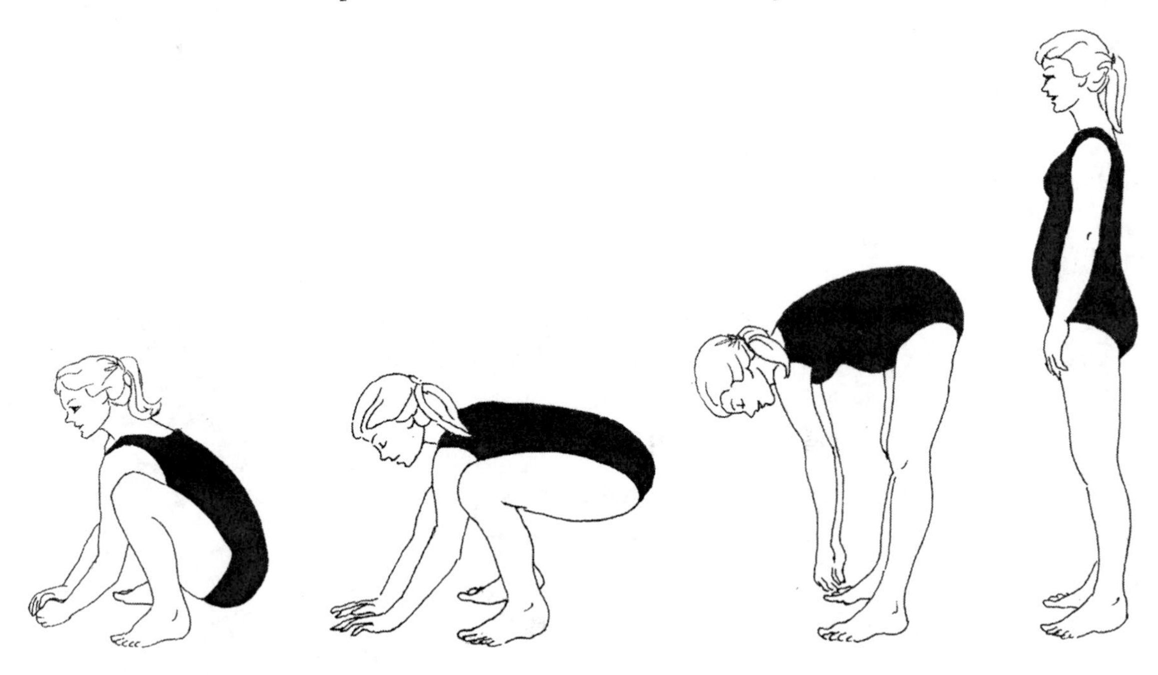

Lifting from a Squat to Protect your Back

Warning: you must not lift any weight from a squat position as you come up from the floor using your back, as was shown in the previous sketches. It is a nice pelvic rock to add but you are using your back for this maneuver. Your back does not need any more weight to lift than the baby in the uterus!

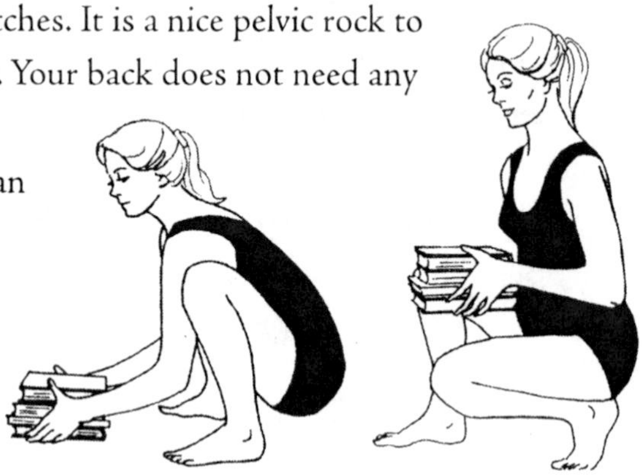

Therefore, when lifting anything heavier than an article of clothing from the floor, use your legs, not your back

It is using simple body mechanics. If you are not pregnant or if you are lifting some weight, use this method of getting up froma squat.

HOW:

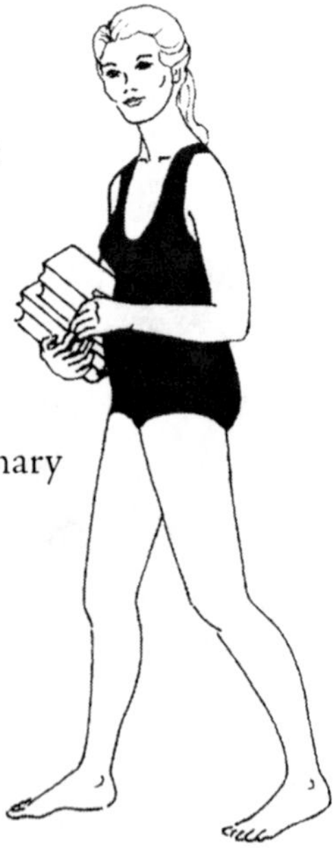

After you are in the squat position, change your posture from the squat to the position with your feet diagonal that is one in front of the other which creates a much larger base and gives you better balance. During pregnancy, women need a broader base to balance their extra weight. It's not an equal distribution and it's concentrated primarily around the expanding uterus. Notice the area of floor if you draw an imaginary square around your feet; compare this area with that of an ordinary squat. Keep your back straight as you use your leg muscles to lift yourself into a standing posture.

Since pregnancy sometimes causes slight dizziness as you change position, a chair or table nearby can be grasped with one hand to steady you. If you are lifting a heavy object remember to use your legs, not your back. As a mother you will be lifting often!

This is also a useful posture for reaching the baby in a crib or bassinet. Use your legs and keep your back straight. No reason to cause extra back strain and discomfort.

WHERE and WHEN:

Squat anytime you find it necessary to reach low: getting into lower cupboards, gardening, picking up laundry or light objects, caring for children, changing diapers, tying shoes, loving, hugging, or talking to a child, helping dress, buttoning, showing things, explaining, the opportunities are endless. Use it often and remember that it is getting you ready for the birth.

Rhondda's AHA

Squatting becomes easier as your pregnancy blooms because the cartilage joints in your pelvis soften to allow the baby through the birth canal in the birth... However, as the baby gets bigger, squatting becomes more difficult as the big uterus is in the way! Start early and be good at it before your tummy gets in the way!

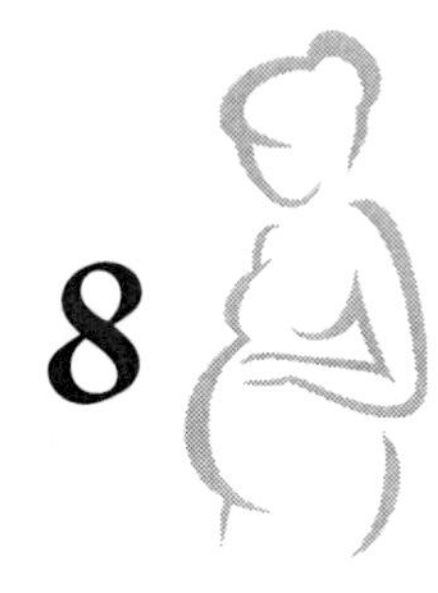

8

The Mysterious Kegel

There isn't a muscle in your body identified as a Kegel—it's named after a gynecologist who discovered that an easy series of "squeezes" within the lower pelvic area of a woman's body had incredible benefits. A huge benefit that every pregnant mother appreciates when Kegel exercises become routine, there is a decreased need to empty the bladder as often with the stronger muscle.

The pubococcygeus muscle is the floor of the pelvis, encompassing the perineal area. As its name indicates, it includes the area from the pubis, in front, to the coccyx, or tailbone, in back. It is the muscle that allows you to control the three openings all women have: the opening from the bladder (urethra), the opening from the uterus (vagina), and the opening from the bowel (rectum).

Try to open or tighten each of these separately and you will find it impossible. They all work together because this one muscle controls the whole area. Your goal is to learn to be conscious of the control of the pubococcygeus muscle, and especially to maintain a constant tension in it. You will call this "Kegeling."

All the organs in the abdomen rest on this layer of muscle. You can imagine how incredibly important that makes it! If it is weak, everything shifts. You could have loss of bladder and bowel control, also your sex life and birth experience would suffer.

Stress incontinence is a result of a weak Kegel muscle.You might experience it in pregnancy. Lots of older women complain of it. That means you have a slight leakage of urine when you sneeze, cough or jump. The best cure and prevention is to regularly do your Kegels for the rest of your life.

The role of the Kegel exercise and muscle is vital during pregnancy, postpartum and for the rest of your life.

Kegeling during Pregnancy, Birth and After Delivery

Most women have learned about the Kegel exercise at some time—few realize how it will affect their lives.

Here is how important it is:

- *During pregnancy,* the extra weight of the uterus stretches the pubococcygeus, which makes exercising it for strength very important. You know that a muscle which is used constantly is able to stretch and return to normal without injury and also is much stronger. A good healthy muscle, having good tone, will be able to support a growing uterus for nine months and return to its usual function and strength after the birth.

- *During the birth process,* the Kegel muscle is put to a great test. It must have enough elasticity to move high into the vaginal wall and not impede the descent of the baby. When you relax this muscle while pushing, you do not slow the birth. If you tighten it during a pushing contraction it will cause discomfort and pain and could slow the progress of labor.

- *After delivery*, the flexing of the Kegel muscle helps healing in general, and episiotomy healing in particular, if an episiotomy was performed. Healing is supported by the increase of blood supply to this area of your body. The same would be true for a tear in the perineum.
- Contracting and relaxing this muscle brings improved circulation to all the tissues in the area. It keeps the muscle healthy and strong to support the abdominal contents.

For the rest of your life, the good condition of this muscle needs to be maintained. The proper alignment of your pelvic and abdominal organs depends ultimately on the Kegel muscle. An improper position, or a sagging or falling of the uterus causes symptoms of backache, heaviness in the pelvis, bladder infections, frequency of urination, incontinence, cystocele and rectocele. These are all problems of aging so keep Kegeling throughout your life. I have purposely listed these unpleasant "women's complaints" because the good tone of your Kegel muscle can prevent them. Use the Kegel to keep everything up and in where it belongs.

Need I remind you about your bonus? Your sexual satisfaction is another good measure of how well you've done your Kegels! By the way, this is a good exercise for men, too.

HOW:

Tighten the "stopping the flow of urine" muscle. Now, as you tighten, pull up or lift with the tightening.

Tighten — lift — lift — hold — let—go.

Count it so that with each tightening you lift to the count of three, hold for one count and relax to the count of two. The whole count takes about two seconds. This will help teach you the constant tension that should be present in this muscle. It should never be completely relaxed while you are awake.

The first times you try this, spread your legs slightly apart, then tighten and release the muscle. Do not allow other muscles to get involved. Buttocks, thighs, and abdomen can be confused at first with the simple Kegel contraction.

Important: your baby will be bouncing about on your bladder. You will need a strong Kegel. You will notice that you do not need to empty your bladder as often with a stronger muscle. Your bathroom visits during the night might decrease, too.

WHERE:

Anywhere—any position. No one should be able to see you using this muscle as long as you are doing it correctly—unless you are like one gal in class who claimed that she could not do the Kegel without opening and closing her mouth, fishlike, at the same time. There really is no physical connection.

Think Kegel ... squeeze and lift!

Talking on the phone is a good time to do twenty. You can brush your teeth and Kegel, watch TV and Kegel, stand in the supermarket line and Kegel, wait for a stoplight and Kegel, hold the door open for children and Kegel, read your emails and Kegel, pelvic rock and Kegel, stir the soup and Kegel, read this and Kegel!!

WHEN:

Twenty times each waking hour for the rest of your life. In other words, only when you are asleep should your Kegel muscle relax.

Rhondda's AHA

Twenty times an hour for the rest of your life!

9

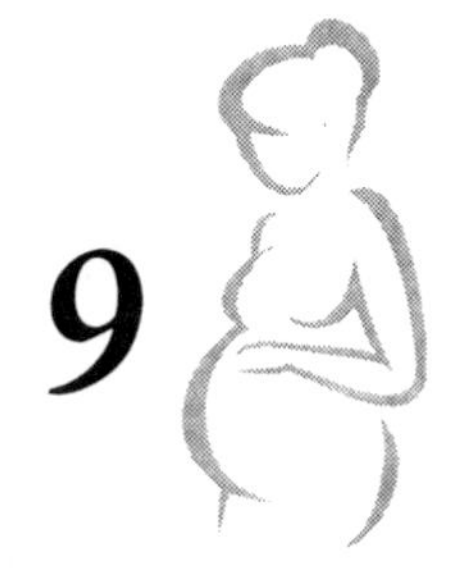

Leg Exercises that Make You Feel Better

The following exercises are offered with circulation of the lower extremities in mind. Use them faithfully and you may have no problems with varicose veins.

Leg elevation is one way of increasing the circulation in the lower part of your body. One good way to elevate your lower body is by raising the foot of your bed with three or four bricks. Your spouse may not like the idea at first, but after a few days you both may find that you are more rested and have lost that "woody" feeling in your legs.

Leg stretches and exercises are critical to your baby. Why?—they keep the circulation active to your uterus. A skimpy supply of blood is not the perfect nourishment for your growing baby.

Keep Your Circulation Moving

Foot Circles and Leg Stretches are easy, fast, and will get your sluggish circulation speeded up. Don't forget that hands-and-knees Pelvic Rock is one of the most important ways of eliminating pelvic pressure on those veins and getting the blood pushed through your circulatory system. I told you that it would be a cure-all.

"When in doubt, do some Pelvic Rocks" is my motto.

Foot Circles Exercises

Since varicose veins can be a threat during pregnancy, this is another good exercise to help minimize that. It makes you feel better and more energetic, too.

By forcing the circulation of blood through your legs, you create an efficient exchange of nutrients and wastes to and from the tissues.

It is better than a walk because the uterus does not become hammered into the pelvis to create pressure, as happens with walking. The good effects of walking when pregnant are somewhat cancelled by the pressure created in the pelvis. So we offer foot circles as an alternative!

HOW:

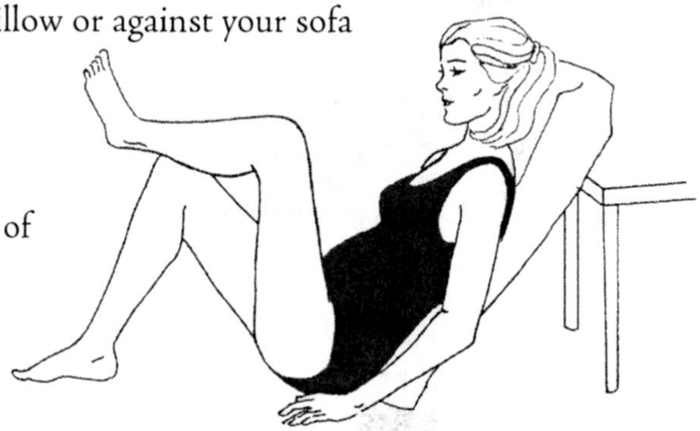

1. Sit on the floor, leaning back against a pillow or against your sofa with your right knee bent.
2. Rest your left ankle on your right knee.
3. Do a series of nine circles to the outside of your foot (clockwise).
4. When you've finished nine circles, your toes are pointing up. Then relax your foot and shake out your whole leg, so that any muscle crampiness is released.
5. Do the same thing with the right ankle resting on the left knee, making counterclockwise circles.
6. Now enjoy the good feeling in your legs and feet.
7. Repeat as much as is comfortable.

Think of tracing the face of a clock with your big toe. Start with your big toe pointing straight up to an imaginary twelve o'clock. Then your toes point to three o'clock, six o'clock, nine o'clock, and then twelve o'clock again. Do three quarter circles, three half circles, three whole circles, all clockwise. Now, do the opposite with the left foot—go counterclockwise.

Here's an added benefit: This will help strengthen the arch in your foot so that you need not be flat-footed with pregnancy.

You can give yourself a muscle cramp in the calf of your leg by pointing your toes. Avoid doing that! Point your heel to relieve the cramp!

WHERE:

Anywhere that you can relax and get into position, you can do foot circles. It's very comfortable to lean against your husband while you do this but a wall or sofa will do.

WHEN:

Do this anytime your legs feel tired. It is especially indicated if you've not rested sufficiently during the day.

You can't control every day the way you'd like, so sometimes a revitalizing exercise is the perfect antidote. It is particularly useful when you have been busy most of the day and have not done enough pelvic rocks, except the standing type which I hope you were able to fit in.

Leg Stretches—Flexing and Extending Ankles and Knees

Not only will leg stretches stimulate circulation in your legs; they will also strengthen your leg muscles and make it easier to carry those extra pounds caused by your growing baby. You may even develop a more shapely leg!

You will be carrying your child for at least a year after he is born, too, so let's get ready now. If you wear high heels, this exercise will help stretch your Achilles tendon, which may have become shortened over the years.

It is a good idea, pregnant or not, to vary the type of heel you wear.

Walking or running barefoot in sand is supposed to be the best exercise for your legs and feet. Sand moves under your feet as you walk to provide a workout for your muscles. Hard floors or cement sidewalks do not "move." Since running barefoot in the sand is not possible for all of us, I've included these easy leg stretches.

HOW:

1. From a tailor sit position, stretch one or both legs away from you at an angle, supporting yourself with your hands.

2. Extend your toes away from you while stretching your leg out straight.

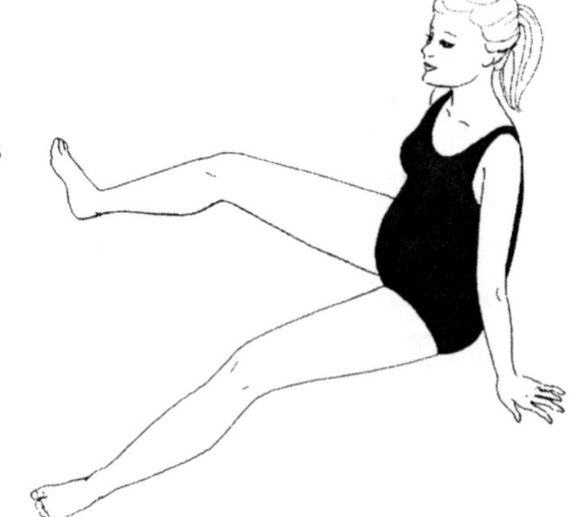

3. Pull your toes toward your body and raise your knee at the same time. The heel will rotate but for maximum effect it should not move from its position. You can do legs separately or together until you feel comfortable. Resume your tailor sitting.

WHERE:

These Leg Stretches can be done anywhere you are tailor sitting on the floor. It is a good way to keep circulation flowing if you sit too long.

WHEN:

They are especially useful when you are involved in an activity and sitting in the tailor sit position. If you feel the need to move but do not wish to interrupt your writing or reading—or simply do not have the energy to move around—this accomplishes the same thing.

Rhondda's AHA

It's easy to think, "I don't have time to do all these things," but what you are saying is, "I don't think it's important enough to take time." You are important and so is your baby in utero, which makes you twice as important.

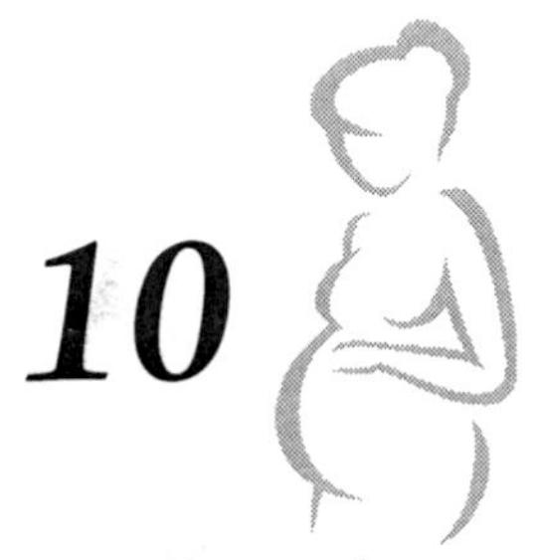

10

Getting Ready for Pushing and Giving Birth

With your expanding girth, it's time to think about the actual process of giving birth to your baby. You will need to begin practicing breath holding for the all-important pushing phase which is the second stage of labor. You also need to learn the ultimate position for giving birth. In *Chapter 7, Squatting Makes the Difference,* you learned to squat … now you need to put that into a position that is also used for the pushing stage of labor.

You are becoming proficient at abdominal breathing. Now let's learn the breathing that will make a difference for your second-stage labor. First let me repeat my "nutshell" review of instructions for natural childbirth.

Natural Childbirth in a Nutshell

1. **In the First Stage of labor,** use abdominal breathing and complete relaxation with each contraction.

2. **In the Second Stage of labor,** take complete, full breaths with each contraction and push as hard as you can while holding your breath.

I know I repeat myself!
You need to be able to say this by heart and with meaning.
It is simple but not always easy!

Breath Holding

It is important that you have a big breath to be able to push properly. Only with full lungs can you push down adequately with your diaphragm. The more usable oxygen you have in your lungs, the longer you can hold your breath and push. The longer you can push without having to replenish your breath, the sooner you will give birth!

However, if you are trying to push after your breath has been used up it will not be working for you. Take a breath when you need more oxygen. That is the only way your pushing will be effective.

Each time you stop pushing to take a breath, the baby slips back in the birth canal. As you reapply the pressure of pushing, the baby descends and forces open the birth canal. Each push is a step forward; when you relax it's a small step back. This is truly hard work. Your body needs enormous amounts of oxygen ... so good, big breaths are necessary for effective pushing.

Learning early to breathe properly for the second stage will greatly improve your efficiency and reduce the time you are in labor.

The position for pushing is very important, too. In a squat position with chin on chest, all your energy is directed toward the baby, helping push the baby through the birth canal. It's as though your back is a bowstring pulled back as far as it will go. The baby is the arrow! The energy of the bowstring gives the power to the arrow. You might not be on your feet in a squat, though that would be ideal, but rather tilted into a forty-five-degree angle, with your arms pulling your legs back, elbows up and out. You will be half sitting, with your coach supporting your shoulders.

As though that is not enough to concentrate on, there is one more thing to remember—relax that baby door, the Kegel muscle. In this position, you can push your baby into the world efficiently and quickly.

HOW:

Tailor sitting posture seems best for practicing this breathing, but whatever position is comfortable for you is fine. The actual position that is used in labor—contour—may be uncomfortable during late pregnancy because the baby is so high up in the abdomen, making breathing very difficult as he pushes into your lungs. When you are actually in second-stage labor, however, the baby has descended very low into the pelvis and in fact is at least partly in the birth canal, so there is plenty of space for the lungs to work properly.

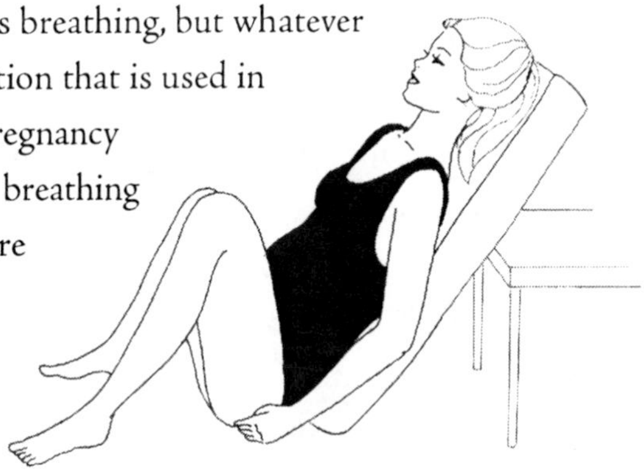

You practice one way and in labor you have another way!

To practice:

1. Sit comfortably in a Tailor position.
2. Take a very large breath, until your lungs feel expanded. Exhale fully.
3. Repeat. You have now taken two large breaths, exhaling each completely.
4. Take another full, deep breath and hold it.
5. Hold as long as the breath lasts—about forty seconds seems a good practice time. (As Dr. Bradley said, "No need for heroics!")
6. When you've held as long as is comfortable, exhale fully.

In Labor:

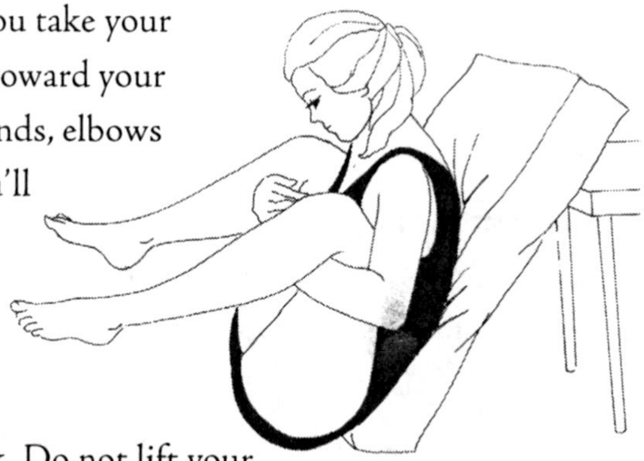

Take the first 2 breaths and blow them out. As you take your third breath, you will also be drawing your knees toward your shoulders and pulling your legs back with your hands, elbows up and out. As you begin holding your breath you'll put your chin to your chest and bear down on the baby with strong, steady pushing. You will be nearly in a squat position, which is the most efficient position for giving birth.

Keep your elbows out, pulling your knees back. Do not lift your tailbone off the bed. You want to push the baby downhill, not uphill. When you have held your breath and pushed as long as is effective, lift your chin off your chest, exhale completely and take another big breath, hold it with chin on chest and keep pushing.

As long as there is a contraction going on, you keep pushing. If you need to do it several times, do it. When the pushing contraction is over, relax and wait for the next. This is extremely hard work but it is also the only way to feel good during a pushing contraction! You will become unaware of the pressure and discomfort as you push hard.

If you feel pain you may not be pushing correctly or hard enough.

You must work with your body. There is nothing to be gained in pushing when the uterus is not in a contraction. Natural Childbirth is simply working with your body when it needs help and staying out of its way when the body does not need any help.

You see how simple this is?

First Stage of Labor: Relax to stay out of the way of your uterus as it contracts. You have no conscious control over the muscles of the cervix which must stretch to open with the pressure of the baby's head. Your job is to relax to stay out of the way of your body. It is the body's natural response to the birth process. You interfere with the process of labor if you do anything but relax during a contraction.

Second Stage of Labor: When the uterus contracts you work with it by pushing. As long as there is a contraction, you push. You do have control of muscles that help get the baby through the birth canal, which is your vagina. The uterus no longer has the full body of your baby completely within it. Pushing helps during a contraction! It also takes away the pain. Push through the pain.

WHEN and WHERE:

During labor, you will use this breathing whenever and wherever you are when you receive that unmistakable urge to push!

Meanwhile, practice daily to improve your breath-holding ability. Have your coach rehearse with you since coaches always hold their breath during your pushes in labor anyway. It's automatic—have you ever tried to breathe normally while watching someone else hold his or her breath? It will give experience in coaching for this final step of labor.

Rhondda's AHA

Practice the breath holding only. Practicing pushing will only contribute to hemorrhoids and is unnecessary, as those muscles are kept strong by your natural body functions, that is, in bowel elimination.

11

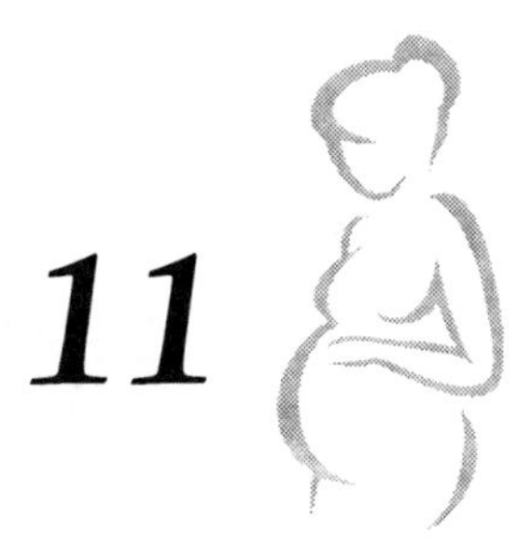

Butterfly or Legs Apart Exercise

When most people think of exercising combined with the word "butterfly" ... swimming is usually the first thing that comes to mind. Not in childbirth. When the butterfly motion in swimming involves the shoulders and arms, in childbirth, it's all about the legs.

The Butterfly or Legs Apart exercise will strengthen the muscles that pull your legs apart. They are weaker than the muscles that pull your legs together. Holding your legs apart is very important during second-stage labor. During labor, your abductors need all the strength they can muster. The added benefit is that your legs will be far stronger post labor when you are up and about.

Not only do you need your legs apart during a push, but between pushes, too, because the baby is low in the birth canal at this time. If your muscles have been completely fatigued with the effort to keep your legs apart during second stage, you may not have enough strength left to support you when you are ready to stand!

Even if you don't walk immediately, you may have trembling, weak legs for several days if you have not prepared. Being proficient with your Butterfly exercise will reduce this.

HOW:

Sit in a comfortable position with knees drawn up and feet together on the floor. Have your husband, partner or coach put their hands on the outside of each of your knees and exert gentle pressure as you push your knees apart as far as they will go. You may change your feet so that the soles are together—it's more comfortable. Bring your knees back together (with no pressure against them) and repeat twice more, with slightly increased pressure each time you spread your knees apart like a butterfly's wings.

Coaching Tips

- It is possible to have more strength in their arms than you do in your legs.
- That will do you no good if you can't practice to build up these muscles so you must teach the rules for this game!
- Some will think that if three times is good, three hundred is better. Not so here. Stiff abductor muscles make every movement painful. Tell your coach to do it only three times! No more.

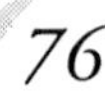

- Also, this muscle, overbuilt, is not pretty, nor is it our objective to have a bulging muscle … just a stronger one.
- Do not put pressure on your knees as you return your legs to the upright, beginning position. This would strengthen the already much stronger adductors—nullifying what we're trying to accomplish.
- And do not let anyone push your knees to the floor as you are spread apart. Ouch!

You do not believe your coach will do any of these things to you, do you? Believe me I have not made them up. They are experiences class members have told me about repeatedly—so I warn you in advance.

WHERE and WHEN:

Wherever and whenever the two of you decide and have the energy to practice. It only takes a few minutes to do three of these once a day. Getting organized to do it will take more time than doing it!

It is worth it as it will have a significant effect on your leg strength post birth.

Rhondda's AHA

One of my fondest memories is carrying our first born out of the delivery room and walking to my hospital room with my husband's arm around me and our baby. The Butterfly exercise can make it possible for you to have that memory, too.

12

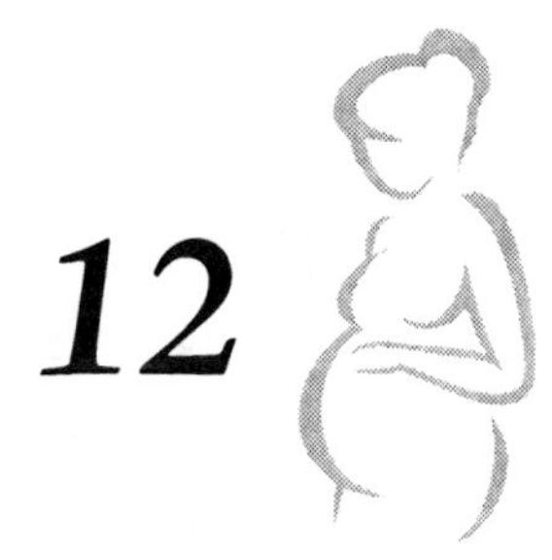

Bust Booster Exercise

The Bust Booster is not only a great preparation for breastfeeding, it is also one of my "lifetime" exercises. It can be used during pregnancy, post-pregnancy and for when the kids are grown and on their own. It will:

1. Strengthen pectoral or chest muscles that help support the breasts.
2. Help to maintain good shoulder posture.
3. Help when you have heartburn and indigestion.
4. Increase blood flow to the breasts; therefore it may be used to increase milk supply.

The pectoral muscles are located beneath and help give support to the breasts. Since the breasts become heavier and bigger with pregnancy and breastfeeding, stronger pectorals are indicated.

Breast tissue is mostly fat deposits surrounding the milk-producing glands and covered by skin. There is no muscle in the breast. This means that breast size cannot be increased by exercise. It also means that breast tissue which sags and stretches cannot be rebuilt—since only muscle tissue can be rebuilt. It is necessary, therefore, to prevent sagging and stretching of breast tissue by good support in a bra. If you prefer to go bra-less, I suggest that you develop a good philosophy about sagging breasts!

The extra weight of your breasts, plus the cuddling position which is frequently used for holding your baby and for breastfeeding, tends to pull your shoulders down. The Bust Booster exercise will help strengthen your chest and shoulders to maintain better posture and at the same time relax these overworked muscles.

HOW:

1. Sit in a tailor position on the floor. Support each breast with the inside of each bent elbow.
2. Press your arms against your body as you raise your hands above your head. This gently massages your breasts, stimulating circulation.
3. Lower your arms until your hands are below your waist, slightly behind you, with palms up.

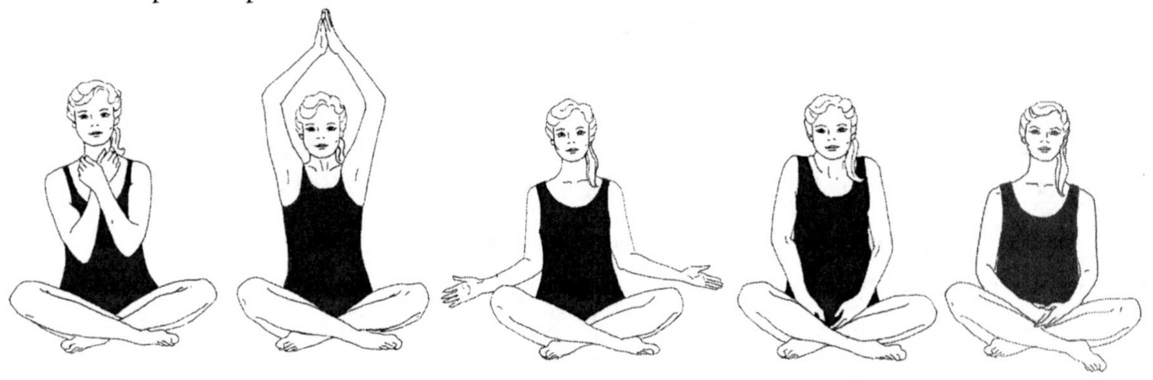

4. Now swing the backs of your hands toward each other, behind you, five times (thumbs up).
5. Bring your hands to your lap.
6. Take a deep breath while trying to touch your shoulders to your ears.
7. Let the breath out and the shoulders drop at the same time, while keeping the breastbone high. It leaves you feeling very good, somewhat invigorated, and with a relaxed upper back.

WHERE:

Do Bust Booster in private, sitting on the floor, and always in a tailor position so that your chest muscles do the work instead of your back.

There are times when steps 6 and 7 can be done to relax your shoulders and upper back without going through the whole exercise. You may need a good stretch in church or in the classroom and this can be done rather unobtrusively. Doing the complete exercise in front of others is sure to create a sensation, however.

WHEN:

During Pregnancy—Do the bust booster approximately three times a day as a chest muscle exercise and to improve your posture. Do it to relax the upper part of your body. It can also be an effective exercise whenever heartburn distress occurs.

After the Birth—Use this for increasing your supply of breast milk, wait and see if you need to do it.

Try to maintain the three times daily to keep muscles in good tone, but if this brings milk rushing out and creates a problem, avoid using it until you are not oversupplied with milk. If you have a need to create a better milk supply, that is, if the baby seems to demand more milk, then try this to hurry up the process. You will find that it is definitely a help!

Rhondda's AHA

You may need a good stretch while working on the computer and this can be the best treatment. Doing the complete exercise will certainly relieve your tired back and chest but if you are in an office you might not want to be that sensational. You will find it feels great. Who cares what anyone thinks!

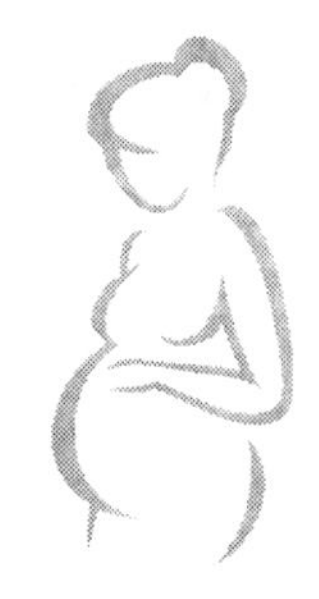

Rhondda's Final Words

Natural Childbirth Exercise Essentials is meant to be a handy, easy guide to your preparation for the birth of your baby. It can be easy to use and to carry with you as you go through your daily life.

It is not an "everything you ever wanted to know about Natural Childbirth!" It is a primer to get you started on the most amazing experience of your life. For a much more complete book about pregnancy and birth please read my book, *Natural Childbirth Exercises for the Best Birth Ever.*

My advice is to also read everything and question everybody. Explore Childbirth as much as you possibly can. This is going to be the most important event in your life. Make it the BEST by making it what you want. Make your own decisions and be informed so that you are making wise choices.

The process of explaining to others what my book is about and why I would be writing it has brought me into focus on what Natural Childbirth is and how important it has been in my life. I began a search into myself to understand what makes some of us embrace it and others to find it abhorrent. I began asking myself, what do we bring to it and what do we receive from it? To you I share my wisdom on the matter.

Natural Childbirth is not just about having a baby.

It is about living your life.

It is about *responsibility.* Accepting it or giving it away.

It is about choices, conviction and completion.

My final Kernel of Truth

I know that to have a Natural Childbirth without drugs you must be *responsible* for it yourself. You cannot expect anyone else to do it for you. Not your coach; not your doctor; not the hospital's staff; and not me nor either of my books. You, and only you, can make it happen. You cannot simply *let* it happen, you must ***make*** it happen.

This is not just about exercising for the birth. No! It is about being responsible for your whole life.

Doing it yourself or letting it be done to you!

When I originally wrote my book, *Natural Childbirth Exercises for the Best Birth Ever,* I thought it was to teach you about Natural Childbirth; to let you know how important it is to do the exercises to prepare your body for a birth without drugs to protect your baby's brain from the harm that can result. I hope I did all that.

But, the idea of being responsible kept repeating in my head.

"If it's to be, It's up to me."

I have lived with my choice of Natural Childbirth for a long time now. I've had enough years to look back over my life and recognize how my choice has influenced and woven through my life. It was a choice that has defined me.

To choose Natural Childbirth is to say:

Let me do it myself.
I can do it by myself; you do not need to do it for me.
Teach me how so I can do it on my own.
Let it not be done to me or for me.
I will make it happen.
Help me, instruct me, coach me, support me, tell me my mistakes but let me do it.
I choose a joyful, exciting , beautiful Natural Childbirth and I will create that experience. Support me in my intention.

Attitude is always an essential ingredient to achieve a Natural Childbirth. Your openness and positivity as you look forward to your birth will greatly enhance your journey through pregnancy.

I see you as a woman who is:

Passionate . . . Strong . . . Capable . . . Sensible . . . Smart . . . Thoughtful!

A woman who is being responsible for your birth and your life! I honor and salute you.

About the Author

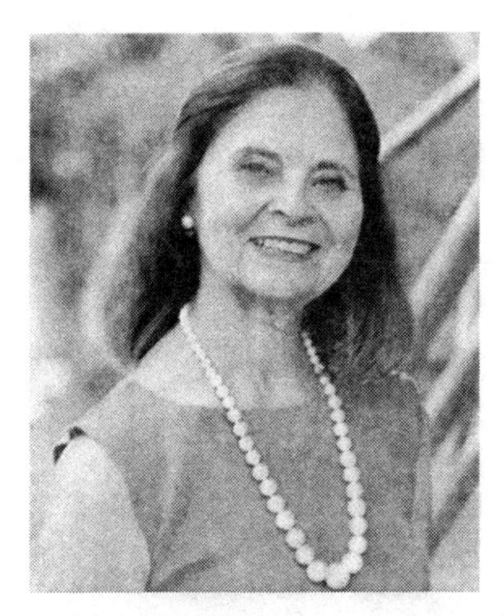

Rhondda Evans Hartman grew up in southern Alberta, Canada where she was a Public Health Nurse before becoming a homemaker and mother. She moved to Colorado after marrying Denver Attorney, Richard E. Hartman in Switzerland while vacationing in Europe. They created five amazing children who have produced nine incredible grandchildren.

She earned her B.S. from the University of Alberta, where she was Vice President of the Student Council in her senior year. She completed her R.N. at the University of Alberta Hospital, School of Nursing in Edmonton, Alberta and became the Public Health Nurse in Lacombe, Alberta. Many years later after all her children were in school, she earned a Master of Arts Degree in Urban Sociology from the University of Colorado in Denver.

For 25 years, she taught classes and trained and supervised other teachers in husband-coached childbirth for Dr. Robert A. Bradley in his Obstetrical Medical Practice in Denver, Colorado. Rhondda is on the Advisory Board of the American Academy of Husband Coached Childbirth, The Bradley Method. She is Charter Member and past president of La Leche League of Colorado and was a meeting leader for many years. Rhondda and Dr. Bradley were frequent speakers at national Natural Childbirth conferences. As an expert on Natural Childbirth exercises, she personally has instructed over 14,000 mothers in having a natural and enjoyable birth. Rhondda has been a guest on national TV in both the United States and Canada.

Natural Childbirth Exercises is her second book. She is also the author of *Exercises for True Natural Childbirth* and is a contributor to the *Five Standards for Safe Childbearing* by David Stewart, PhD. and *Compulsory Hospitalization or Freedom of Choice in Childbirth?* by Stewart and Stewart, editors.

Contact Rhondda through her website:

www.NaturalChildbirthExercises.com

Follow Rhondda and Natural Childbirth Exercises on:

Twitter: @BirthExercises

https://www.facebook.com/NaturalChildbirthExercises

Pinterest: Natural Childbirth Exercises – Rhondda Hartman

Blog: http://NaturalChildbirthExercises.com/blog

LinkedIn Group: Natural Childbirth Exercises

To have a natural and joyful birth experience you must learn this technique:

Stay Calm.
Breathe deeply.
Acknowledge what is happening in your body.
Rise above it.
Know that in a minute's time it is going to go away.
Rest in between.
Get ready for it to start again.

Do this until you get that unmistakable urge to push.
Then push with all your strength to greet your newborn babe.
Learn this Technique.
I am not telling you it is easy.
I am telling you it is possible.

Rhondda Evans Hartman, Author
Natural Childbirth Exercises for the Best Birth Ever
and ***Natural Childbirth Exercise Essentials***

BUY THE BOOKS!

YES, I want ___ autographed copies of *Natural Childbirth Exercise Essentials*: $12.99 plus $6.00 shipping

YES, I want ___ autographed copies of *Natural Childbirth Exercises*: $25.00 plus $6.00 shipping

YES, I want ___ autographed copies of both books: $28.50 (a 25% discount) plus $8.50 shipping

For 10 copies or more, call Rhondda for a deal at 303-789-0320

Also, books may be ordered at *NaturalChildbirthExercises.com*

YES, I am interested in having Rhondda Evans Hartman speak to my company, association, or organization. Please send me information.

Include $6 for shipping and handling for one book, and $2.50 for each additional book. Colorado, Ohio and New York residents must include applicable sales tax. Canadian or other foreign orders must include payment in US funds with 7% GST added.

Payment must accompany orders. Allow 3 weeks for delivery.

My check or money order of $___________ is enclosed.

Please charge my   Visa   MasterCard   American Express   Discover

Name____

Organization____

Address____

City/State/Zip____

Phone_________________________ Email_______________________

Card #____

Exp.Date______________________ CVV code____________________

Signature____

Make your check payable and return to:

Parkland Press, Ltd. • 3755 S. Broadway • Englewood, CO 80110

CPSIA information can be obtained
at www.ICGtesting.com
Printed in the USA
FFOW01n0538170616
25083FF

9 780988 411005